$AVING MONEY
ON SENIOR CARE

How to Make Aging Affordable

Ryan Malone

A Note to the Reader

This publication is designed to provide competent and reliable information, however, it is sold with the understanding that the author and publisher are not in any way rendering legal, financial or other professional advice. Laws and practices vary by state and may change from the time this publication was written and/or published. If legal or other expert assistance is required, please seek the services of a professional. The author and publisher also do not endorse any source cited in this publication. The author and publisher specifically disclaim any and all liability that is incurred in connection with the content of this book.

Saving Money on Senior Care: How to Make Aging Affordable is copyrighted by Ryan Malone and SmartBug Media, Inc. No portion of this book may be reprinted or reproduced in any way without express written permission.

SmartBug Media, Inc.
2549-B Eastbluff Drive
#417
Newport Beach, CA 92660
info@smartbugmedia.com

Editor: Ryan Malone
Self-publishing & Design Partners: Studio 6 Sense | studio6sense.com

DEDICATION

To my beautiful wife and daughter:
Every day with you makes me smile more brightly
than I ever thought possible.

CONTENTS

ONE

WHY WE NEED
THIS BOOK

She Was Strong. I Was Lucky.

My father died at the age of 52 in 1989. Seemingly aware of the likelihood of his early demise, my father had made basic arrangements for my mother through a life insurance policy. He was also lucky enough to be of the generation that we received a pension from his former employer. At the age of 58, my mother's financial future had been diligently planned.

My mother is a strong woman – sometimes too strong. I had just turned 17 when my father died. He'd been in the hospital for more than six months after a failed heart bypass surgery. I was at summer basketball camp when I was called into the coaches' office for a call from my mother. I knew how the conversation would go.

Mom did a wonderful job. She finished raising me and had the strength to smile when I drove away to college a year later. I could see her crying in my rearview mirror, but she didn't let it show while I was there. It was all smiles and good wishes.

She built a wonderful support network of friends, family and local business leaders. She served as president for several women's clubs in her San Diego County city and became an influencing voice in local politics. I was so very proud of her. We were proud of each other.

She planned for what she thought were all the possible scenarios. She meticulously created a budget that would enable her to maintain a good lifestyle and her home well into her eighties. She also planned for death, putting in place her will, trust, advanced healthcare directive and power of attorney documents for medical and finances.

She was all set, right?

Wrong.

What she didn't plan for was what so many millions of older Americans neglect to plan for – long-term care. In her parents' generation, she was. In his book *Caring for Our Parents*, Howard Gleckman notes that healthcare advances have changed the way people age. It used to be that people got old, they got sick and they passed away. Complications from pneumonia or even a broken leg were often fatal. Today, healthcare has extended life spans, but often at a quality of life that requires outside assistance, frequent medical treatments and a benefits support system that is not able to support its citizens.

The intent of the comment above is not to be taken as a cold-hearted concern about cost. In fact, we enjoy many more years with our loved ones – more memories, more smiles and more tears. But everything comes at cost. And many experts say the two most expensive things in your life are your house and elder care. My family knows first hand the truth of this reality.

July 7, 2005

In 2005, my mother had a stroke. I was 33.

That a 73-year old woman had a stroke is not unusual. Mom's case was unique because of the series of complications that nearly killed her. In the eighteen months following her stroke, she required back surgery to remove a staph infection from her spine, a perforated intestine that required stomach surgery, several MRSA infections requiring IV antibiotics and a broken hip. She spent several weeks in the surgical intensive care unit recovering from her back surgery. Many of these nights, I feared the worst, but my mom's a fighter.

The medical system these days isn't a big fan of keeping people in the hospital. They're highly trained at treating acute problems and dealing with specific injuries and conditions. In fact, we have some of the most skilled doctors in the world.

But when you're older and it comes to recovery from serious illness, your options are usually to go home or go to a skilled nursing facility where they can provide some therapy, administer IVs and other things requiring a registered nurse.

During this time, she spent nearly six months back and forth between the hospital and skilled nursing. In January of 2006, I moved Mom from San Diego, California to Orange County (right between San Diego and Los Angeles) and from skilled nursing to assisted living.

When Mom arrived in assisted living, she could not stand or walk and required a 24-hour caregiver. She could not eat or drink on her own and was in a deep state of depression. Through a lot of love and hard work on her part, she attended my wedding a little over a year later.

Mom required a live-in caregiver for many years to assist with activities of daily living and medication. She now lives in assisted living and is doing pretty well - all things considered.

Mom did not have long-term care insurance, supplemental health insurance or anything other than her HMO, which she later transitioned to Medicare and a supplemental health insurance plan through AARP.

Whether you are facing immediate long-term care financial pressures, or you are planning for the future, I've written this book to provide guidance and teach. It will expose you to the pros and cons of the many different ways to pay for elder care expenses.

Consider it your toolbox as your build your elder care financial strategy.

How to Use This Book

I've read many financial books on senior care and spoken to hundreds of providers. They all mean well, but I've never found one that accomplished these two things:

1. Gave families a broad perspective of the different ways to pay for elder care

2. Provided guidance about what to look for and what not to get caught by

The latter is so important. When our parents need additional care, we are placed under enormous pressure to make the right decision. As a result, marketing becomes very effective, and we are often attracted to messaging and claims that would have otherwise been ineffective. This book both educates and protects you, helping you to make the best decision with the most possible information.

Each chapter discusses a different financing option. The chapters are arranged in the same general outline:

- What it is

- How it works

- Who's it for

- Who's it **not** for

- Some examples

- What to look for in a provider

- Things to be careful of when choosing a provider

I sincerely hope you enjoy the book, and that it provides you with enough information to have a productive conversation with whomever you decide to use for elder care financing. As always, please don't hesitate to share your comments or questions with me at ryan@insideeldercare.com.

Be strong,
Ryan Malone

LONG-TERM CARE INSURANCE

How concerned are you about being able to provide care or financial assistance for a parent?

This question, asked of 500 baby boomers between the ages of 42 and 61, revealed that 48% of them are indeed "concerned" about their ability to provide care for an aging parent.[1]

According to a 2005 report by the Pew Research Center, there are 10 million baby boomers raising kids while simultaneously providing financial support to an aging parent. Also known as the "sandwich generation," many boomers experience financial and emotional strain under the pressure of supporting both their children and their parents.

Naturally, our loved ones will reach a time in their lives when they may find that they are less agile, less healthy, and perhaps less able. You may be faced with this predicament when it comes to your parents, or even your siblings or spouse.

It is not surprising that health-care costs in general are a major expense for most seniors. But what can really impose a financial burden on families is when a senior needs day-to-day care. According to 2006 data from the MetLife Mature Market Institute, the average annual cost for an assisted-living facility which helps relatively healthy seniors with daily activities, such as eating and bathing, is $35,616. Meanwhile, the average cost of a private room at a nursing home is $75,190 a year. In larger cities, like New York or Stamford, nursing home costs can exceed $100,000 a year. Unfortunately, Medicare

---

1 http://www.usatoday.com/money/industries/health/2007-06-24-elderly-care-poll_N. htm?loc=interstitialskip

doesn't cover most daily care costs, but the good news is that with some advance planning, there are a number of ways to manage these expenses.

Your loved ones may have elected to purchase *long-term care insurance* for themselves when they were in their 50s or 60s. When the time is right, you can contact your LTCI representative to initiate a claim.

For those of you who are thinking ahead regarding long-term care insurance for a parent or for yourself, here are some of the details should know.

What is Long Term Care Insurance?

Long-term care insurance (LTC or LTCI) is an insurance product that covers the cost of long-term care not covered by health insurance, Medicare, or Medicaid.

Many individuals who require long-term care are not suffering from a particular ailment, but instead, they are unable to perform the basic activities of daily living (ADLs) such as dressing, bathing, eating, medication management or toileting. Some have problems with mobility or cognitive impairments like Alzheimer's or other forms of dementia.

Age alone is not a determining factor in needing long-term care. About 60% of individuals over age 65 will require at least some type of long-term care services during their lifetime. Surprisingly, about 40% of those receiving long-term care today are between 18 and 45. While the information in this chapter still applies to those individuals, our discussion will focus particularly on the needs of seniors.

Many people buy long-term care insurance because the options it provides gives them peace of mind as they age. Long-term care insurance offers several advantages to policyholders:

- Provides a wider range of caregiver options

- Protects your assets, financial independence and standard of living

- Allows you to receive care at home

- Provides a substantial yet flexible safety net for their future well-being

What are Activities of Daily Living (ADLs)?

The degree to which an individual requires help performing ADLs determines the person's needed level of care, and thus, the cost of care. There are six categories of ADLs:

- Hygiene (bathing, grooming, shaving and oral care)
- Continence
- Dressing
- Eating (the ability to feed oneself)
- Toileting (the ability to use a restroom)
- Transferring (actions such as going from a seated to standing position and getting in and out of bed)

There's another category of activities known as IADLs, or instrumental activities of daily living. These are more subtle and complex social activities and can include:

- Finding and utilizing resources (looking up phone numbers, using a telephone, making and keeping doctor's appointments)
- Driving or arranging travel (either by public transportation or personal vehicle)
- Preparing meals (opening containers, using kitchen equipment)
- Shopping (getting to stores and purchasing necessities like food or clothing)
- Doing housework (doing laundry, maintaining a clean living space)
- Managing medication (taking prescribed dosages at correct times and keeping track of medications)
- Managing finances (basic budgeting, paying bills and writing checks)

Many seniors who live independently can perform most or all IADLs sufficiently, but difficulty performing any one of them can indicate that long-term care is needed.

How Does Long-Term Insurance Work?

When you buy LTCI, you are really buying a bucket of money to be used in the event you require care outside of health insurance, Medicare and Medicaid. LTCI policies have similar variables that determine your premium and benefits. They include:

- Daily benefit amount

- Benefit period

- Elimination period

- Home care benefit

- Inflation protection

When considering each variable, keep in mind the factors that could impact the overall cost of your policy:

- Health

- Age

- Marital status

- The benefits you choose

- Any discounts you may qualify for

Daily Benefit

The daily benefit is the maximum dollar amount that the insurance company must pay for your care on any given day. Some policies pay benefits on a weekly or monthly basis, but the total benefit is calculated using a per-day amount.

The daily benefit can range from $40 to $500 per day depending on the carrier. The maximum daily benefit is typically allocated for a stay in a skilled nursing facility, whereas policies may differ on the portion of the daily benefit available for assisted living communities and home care.

Benefit Period

The *benefit period* is the *maximum* amount of time that you will receive benefits. The benefit period is expressed in years, and can range from one year to unlimited, lifetime coverage.

The lifetime maximum is usually calculated by multiplying the benefit period by the daily benefit amount. For example, if you purchased a three-year benefit period with a daily benefit of $100, your lifetime maximum would be $109,500 (1,095 days times $100).

Elimination Period

The *elimination period* is the length of time in which you must pay out-of-pocket for long-term care services *before* the insurance policy begins paying benefits. This is similar to a deductible in traditional health care plans.

Elimination periods range from zero days to as many as 730 days (2 years). As with medical insurance, the longer your elimination period (i.e., a higher deductible), the lower your premiums will be. However, the elimination period can create a risky situation for many people since they are responsible for all expenses during that period. This is in contrast to traditional medical insurance deductibles where you have a dollar amount deductible.

Warning: do NOT underestimate the cost of medical care when you choose the elimination period. It is costly and likely to become more costly.

Home Care Benefits

Home care benefits allow the policyholder to receive daily care at home — and since many people prefer the comfort and familiarity of their own home, this is an important benefit to consider. This benefit can include skilled professionals, home health aides, personal care attendants, homemaker services and adult day care.

Inflation Protection

Inflation protection is a common option with most LTCI policies. Offered as either compound or simple inflation protection, these riders protect against the rising cost of healthcare. Inflation riders are designed to increase your benefit while keeping your premiums level for the life of your policy.

Most inflation riders are offered at 5%. A compound inflation rider will double every 14.6 years, whereas a simple inflation rider will double every 20 years. The decision of which one to choose should be based on expected lifespan.

Types of Policies

There are three types of policies: *comprehensive, facility-only,* and *home care-only.* Some carriers only offer *comprehensive* policies, and no longer provide *facility-only* or *home care-only.*

Comprehensive LTCI policies offer benefit features for many types of care:

- Nursing Home Facilities
- Assisted Living Facilities (including Alzheimer facilities)
- Home care
- Adult day care
- Respite care
- Care coordination

Payment of Benefits

Most policies pay benefits by reimbursing policyholders for expenses incurred, up to a pre-determined amount. If the reimbursement amount is less than the maximum daily amount, the remaining funds can be used in the future. For instance, if you have a 3-year policy with a $100 daily benefit and your incurred expense is $50, the policy will pay out for 6 years until funds run out.

Discounts Available

As with auto or homeowners insurance, insurance companies often provide discounts if you have many personal policies through the same carrier. A healthy couple can often receive a 10-40% discount from what they would pay if they used a separate carrier for LTCI.

Who's a Good Fit for Long-Term Care Insurance

Unlike some of the other financial options we'll discuss in this book, there are no age requirements to purchase LTCI. However, age and health are the primary factors that impact insurability and the cost of the policy. The best time to buy long-term care insurance is between the ages of 45 to 55 before you have a medical condition that could impact premiums.

Cost of Delaying LTCI

Waiting to purchase LTCI has several negative financial impacts:

- Premiums rise every year that you age

- As the cost of healthcare increases, you will require a larger benefit and pay higher premiums

- You risk developing a medical issue that could impact your insurability

It is a common misconception that waiting to buy LTCI will save money on premiums. Unfortunately, LCTI premiums rise as you age much in the same way that life insurance premiums do.

Who Long-Term Care Insurance is Not For

Although there are no age limitations, LTCI is not for everyone. Individuals in the following situations may not be good candidates:

- Individuals with an existing medical condition likely to require additional care

- Individuals who currently receive Medicaid benefits

- Those whose only income is social security

- Low-income individuals who would spend a large percentage of their income on insurance premiums

Example: 50-Year-Old Male

Consider this scenario: a 50-year-old gentleman purchases a comprehensive LTCI policy that includes $150 daily benefit, four-year benefit period, 90-day elimination period, and inflation protection with a major carrier.

The policyholder is currently paying an annual premium of $1,338.75, or just over $111.00 per month. If he owned the policy until he was 85 years old, he would have paid in a total of $46,856.25 in premiums.

But, if he had waited five years to purchase the same policy, the annual premium would be $1,974.37. The increased premium takes into account that he's now five years older and also reflects the increase in care costs. If he owned the policy until he was 85 years old he would have paid in a total of $59,231.10.

Waiting five years to purchase his LCTI policy would have cost him an extra $12,374.85 in premiums over his lifetime. It certainly didn't save him any money, and he was also uninsured for five years!

Ten Tips for Buying Long-Term Care Insurance

1. **Where do you want to retire?** Research the average daily cost of care in the area which you are planning to retire to help you determine an appropriate daily benefit amount.

2. **How much retirement income will you receive?** The more discretionary income you have, the lower the daily benefit you may need to purchase.

3. **Extra costs to think about.** A private room in a skilled nursing facility versus the actual cost of an assisted living community could be greater than the average costs in a region.

4. **Consider your family health history.** If you have a family history of Alzheimer's or simply longevity, you may want to consider policies that cover longer periods of care such as unlimited policies, joint policies for married couples or policies with 5 – 8 year benefit periods. Some Alzheimer's patients have been known to require care for more than 20 years.

5. **Consider your assets.** The greater your nest egg, the longer the elimination period you can get by with. The recommended maximum elimination is 90 days. Although several carriers offer elimination periods up to 730 days, the reduction in premiums does not offset the significant increase in your share of the upfront costs past 90 days.

6. **Start planning early.** The younger you are, the more important it is to consider the future cost of your elimination period (deductible), since the cost of long-term care is expected to increase with inflation. It may be more cost effective over the long run to select a shorter elimination period.

7. **Do you want to receive care at home?** If the home care benefit is a priority, seriously consider a reduced elimination period for the home care portion.

8. **Beware of low cost policies!** Sometimes it is true that you get what you pay for — make sure that the insurance carrier has a strong history in the LTCI market that you can review for premium stability and claims payment experience. Policies that are priced significantly below market can end up costing you more in the long run.

9. **Age and inflation:** When considering inflation protection, consider your age. If you are 70 years or older, a 5% simple rider (increase) may be sufficient. If you are younger than 70, a compound 5% rider makes more sense because it will increase the benefit amount faster and to a greater degree in the long run.

10. **Overall affordability is critical** when designing your LTCI plan. A conservative policy could change your family's life when needed. As a rule of thumb, a "short and fat" policy (e.g., a 3-year policy with $180 daily benefit) is almost always more advantageous than a "lean and long" policy (e.g., a 6-year policy with $90 daily benefit).

What to Watch Out For

Long-term care insurance is desirable because it puts the policyholder in the driver's seat and offers myriad options depending on your needs. With that in mind, here are some important things to watch out for when designing your policy.

Inflation Protection

The cost of care has been increasing about 5% every year. Some companies choose not to promote inflation coverage but rather offer their customers policies that follow the consumer price index. This only amounts to a 3% inflation clause and does not provide enough protection against rising care costs. Note: most healthcare costs have risen at a rate far higher than inflation for the past few years.

Insurance Agent, Financial Planner, or LTCI Broker?

If you don't already work with an insurance carrier, consider purchasing your policy from only a reputable LTCI *broker* rather than a financial advisor or general insurance agent. Brokers can often provide access to multiple carries. Since an LTCI broker does not have a contract with any one insurance carrier, they will be more likely to shop around on your behalf. Brokers are a good check and balance for the quote you'll receive from your carrier.

Be cautious in regard to *regional* carriers. It is often more difficult to assess the reputation of small LTCI carriers. Stick with larger, nationwide firms who may have stronger balance sheets.

Do some research: check the insurance company's financial ratings, how long they've been in business and the size of their LTCI portfolio. A quick Internet search can yield a lot of valuable information about a company's premium stability and payout history.

The Elimination Period

If home care is important to you, select a short elimination period. Most policyholders not only open claims at home several months after care is needed, but they also make the mistake of selecting a 30-90 day elimination period. This delay creates a tremendous financial burden that could have been avoided.

Be sure to ask if the elimination period you select is a one-time period, or if it repeats itself each time you make a new claim. Policy waivers are available, so that homecare is available from the very first day. But if you find that extra cost is not affordable for you, then shorten the elimination period as much as possible.

Don't Underestimate Health Concerns

Once you have purchased a policy you are happy with, take advantage of the benefits you are entitled to when a health situation arises. It's easy for a wife to care for a husband for "just one more day" which could turn into weeks or months. Many times, a "temporary" health condition turns into something that requires long-term care. Avoid the tendency to underestimate the care you may need by assuming that the health issue is minor or temporary. Even if you are in doubt, it never hurts to contact your broker to initiate a claim. If the claim is approved, you can then decide if you want to use the policy.

Calendar Days vs. Paid Days

Policies can be written in terms of *calendar days* or *paid days*. This could make a huge difference in your out-of-pocket expenses for home health care. Shop around and read the fine print.

For example, consider a policy with a 90-day elimination period. It is easy to assume that means 90 *calendar days*. **Rather, the policy is written so that it's 90 *paid* days that count.**

Let's say your initial home care involves a visit from a care agency three days a week. This means you actually only accrue *3 days of credit per week* towards the 90-day period. If that goes on for some time, it would require 30 weeks of home care to satisfy the requirement of 90 daily service visits. In this case, you may recover before you fulfill the elimination period, and thus will not be reimbursed by the insurance company for the care you paid for out-of-pocket.

A policy based on *calendar days* is a far more advantageous option. An even better policy upgrade offers ways to reduce your elimination period to zero days for home care.

Geriatric Care Management

Care management companies can help families track and control costs. Most policies only cover the initial assessment, but the on-going costs of geriatric care management are often not covered. Be aware of your policy limitations and benefits in this area.

Be Selective About Bells and Whistles

Again, shop around and read the fine print. Insurance companies may try to offer added-value features beyond the basic benefits, but most of them don't add much value at all. Be thoughtful and realistic about your needs and priorities when considering additional benefits.

However, there are a few added features however, that may be worth considering. The *waiver for home care,* the *shared care rider for a couple,* and *survivor benefits* are a few examples.

Questions To Ask a Prospective LTCI Broker

Be thorough about finding an LTCI broker you trust. First, visit your state's Department of Insurance website to verify if an agent is in good standing and validly licensed for all the carriers stated. Here are some questions you may want to ask prospective brokers when shopping around:

1. Do you *specialize* in long-term care insurance? If so, how long have you specialized in LTCI?

2. Are you licensed to sell partnership policies? [if applicable in your state]

3. Do you own a long-term care policy yourself?

4. Are you licensed to sell more than a single carrier?

5. Can you provide comparable and competitive quotes from other carriers? (Although an agent is licensed by one carrier, they are sometimes able to sell other policies. However, they usually receive higher commissions for selling their carrier's products.)

What is a Partnership Policy?

The Long-term Care Insurance Partnership Program was developed jointly by states and private insurance companies in the 1980s to lessen individuals' reliance on Medicaid to finance their LTCI. Individuals who purchase qualifying policies first rely on their private insurance benefits before accessing Medicaid benefits to cover LTC costs. The individual may still qualify for Medicaid *provided they meet certain income and asset criteria.*

Questions to Ask About the Policy

1. Does the policy qualify for the LTCI Partnership Program in your state?

2. If you are under the age of 70: Does the policy include a rider

for automatic 5% compound inflation protection while the premium remains level?

3. Does the policy pay the same daily rate for home care and assisted living as it does for a skilled nursing facility?

4. Can I hire a non-licensed person for homemaker services at home?

5. Is the elimination period for home care benefits defined by paid days or calendar days? (As discussed above, calendar days are more beneficial.)

6. Do your own cost research by visiting local facilities and contacting home care agencies. Is your daily benefit enough to cover the cost of your preferences?

7. What are the financial ratings of the insurance company? ("A" ratings are preferable.)

8. How long has the company been selling LTCI? (Preferably the portfolio is at least 15 years old.)

9. Does the company have a history of premium increases on any of the LTCI policies after they have been sold? (Preferably no more than oncewhich should be given to you in writing.)

10. For policies that offer a temporary premium rate guaranty (e.g., 5 years): What happens if a premium increase on the portfolio occurred during my guaranty period? Will I be subject to the same increase when the guaranty expires, or is my policy protected until the next increase?

Long-term care insurance is a great way to prepare for the future – but it may not be something you can use immediately to solve more pressing eldercare funding issues. The following chapters explore other options for families facing the high cost of eldercare today.

What about the CLASS Act?

Incorporated in the Healthcare reform bill passed shortly before the end of 2009 is the CLASS Act. The acronym stands for Community Living Assistance Services and Supports Act. The CLASS act essentially establishes a national long-term care insurance program designed to help seniors and the disabled pay for in-home care. While the CLASS may become an alternative to private long-term care insurance, it is not clear at the time of this writing exactly how the program will be implemented.

Special Thanks

I would like to thank Jody Hubbard for her expert contributions in this chapter. Jody is an independent insurance broker in San Diego county and a long-time advocate for seniors. Jody can be reached at:

Jody Hubbard
Long Term Care Insurance Services
2033 Elijo Avenue, #590
Cardiff, CA 92007
Toll – free (866)944-3800
www.hubbardltc.com
info@hubbardltc.com

Need a Provider in Your State?

Inside Elder Care maintains a list of long-term care insurance providers nationwide. For a list of long-term care insurance providers in your state, visit www.insideeldercare.com/LTC.

REVERSE MORTGAGES

Many seniors today own their own home outright, having purchased it when prices were extremely low. Even if they don't have clear title to the property, their existing mortgage could be small enough to be paid off in full, making a reverse mortgage worthwhile. Consider this scenario: a house purchased in 1974 for $22,000 could now be worth at least ten times that amount. Dipping into home equity to fund eldercare may be a sensible solution for your family. Let's explore the ins-and-outs of this option to see if it's the right choice for your family.

What is a Reverse Mortgage?

A reverse mortgage is a loan for seniors that allows them to convert their home equity into cash. The homeowner is not obligated to repay the loan for as long as the home is their principal residence. You, or the last borrower, must repay the loan (plus interest) when the homeowner dies, sells the property, or fails to live in the home for 12 consecutive months — in the case of a nursing home stay, for instance.

For the purposes of this book, I will focus on Home Equity Conversion Mortgages (HECM loans) which are federally-insured reverse mortgages underwritten by the U.S. Department of Housing and Urban Development (HUD) and the Federal Housing Administration (FHA). HECM loans are widely available, have no income or medical requirements and the proceeds can be used for any purpose.[1]

The HECM program is designed to help the borrower make an informed decision about whether this type of loan is right for them.

---

1 Additionally, your state may offer two other types of reverse mortgages: **single-purpose reverse mortgages** which are offered by some state and local government agencies and nonprofit organizations and **proprietary reverse mortgages** which are loans backed by private companies.

Prior to applying, you will be required to meet with an HECM counselor who will discuss costs, financial implications and possible alternatives.

How the HECM Works

As mentioned above, the HECM program allows seniors age 62 and above to borrow funds from their home equity, and they are not obligated to repay the debt as long as they live in their home. Unlike ordinary home equity loans, a FHA reverse mortgage HECM does not require repayment as long as the home is your principal residence. Lenders recover their principal plus interest when the home is sold. The remaining value of the home is dispensed to you or your heirs. You can never owe more than your home's value.

Reverse mortgage loans are *non-recourse loans*, meaning that if the sales proceeds are insufficient to pay the amount owed, FHA will pay the lender the amount of the shortfall. FHA collects an insurance premium from all borrowers to provide this coverage.

An adjustable rate program from the HECM offers five payment plans:

- **Tenure** - equal monthly payments as long as at least one borrower lives and continues to occupy the property as a principal residence.

- **Term** - equal monthly payments for a fixed period of months selected.

- **Line of Credit** - unscheduled payments or in installments, at times and in an amount of your choosing until the line of credit is exhausted

- **Modified Tenure** - combination of line of credit plus scheduled monthly payments for as long as you remain in the home

- **Modified Term** - combination of line of credit plus monthly payments for a fixed period of months selected by the borrower

Borrowers may change their payment plan for a small fee. If you chose a Fixed Rate program, the only payment option is a full withdrawal. (Program rates and options are subject to change).

During the term of a reverse mortgage loan, the borrower makes no monthly payments on their traditional mortgage. Thus, as your debt grows, your equity is lessened. But remember, a reverse mortgage is a non-recourse loan; you cannot owe more than your home's value at the time the loan is repaid. Any shortfall is paid for by the federal insurance program that is paid by all HECM borrowers must purchase.

When you decide to take out a reverse mortgage, you *must* pay off the existing mortgage. You may qualify for a reverse mortgage even if you still owe money on an existing mortgage, but the reverse mortgage must be in a first lien position, so any existing debt must be paid off. You can pay off the existing mortgage with the proceeds from the reverse mortgage or money from your savings.

Reverse mortgage borrowers continue to own their homes, so they are still responsible for property taxes, insurance, and repairs. If you fail to carry out these responsibilities, your loan could become due and payable in full.

How Much Money You Can Get

The amount you can borrow depends on your age, the current interest rate, other loan fees and the appraised value of your home or FHA's HECM mortgage limit for your area, whichever is less.

Naturally, the more valuable your home is, the older you are and the lower the interest, the more you are able to borrow. If there is more than one owner, the age of the youngest owner is used to determine the amount you can borrow. For an estimate of HECM cash benefits based on your age, home value and current interest rate, use one of the online calculators listed in the side bar.

Online Calculators – A Great Place to Start

HUD recommends these helpful tools:

AARP Reverse Mortgage Calculator
http://rmc.ibisreverse.com//rmc_pages/rmc_aarp/aarp_index.aspx

National Reverse Mortgage Lenders Association Calculator
http://rmc.ibisreverse.com/default_nrmla.aspx

There are no asset or income criteria for a HECM. In addition, there is no limit on the value of homes qualifying for a HECM. The value of your home will be determined by an appraisal. However, your borrowing limit is determined by the appraised value or the current FHA HECM mortgage limit of $625,500—whichever is lower. You are charged an upfront insurance premium of 2 percent of the maximum claim amount that may be borrowed plus a 0.5 percent annual premium.

An HECM loan cannot exceed the existing federal lending limit that is currently $625,000. Should you pursue an HECM loan, your HUD-approved counselor will be able to clarify the current lending limit.

Advantages of Reverse Mortgages

- Allows the homeowner to remain in the home permanently

- Pays off existing mortgages on the home

- Simple to qualify for because credit score and income are not factors

- No monthly payments are due for as long as the home is the principal residence

- The homowner receives payments on flexible terms: as a credit line for emergencies, monthly, as a lump sum, or any combination of these

- Heirs are able to keep the remaining home equity after the balance of the loan is paid off

- Proceeds are tax-exempt

- In some states, a three-day right to cancel offers borrowers an opportunity to change their minds

Basic Facts on Reverse Mortgages

Borrower Requirements:

- 62 years of age or older
- Must own and use the property as a primary residence
- Must pay property taxes and homeowners' insurance
- Must not be delinquent on any federal debt
- Must participate in a consumer information session given by an approved HECM counselor

Loan Amount is Based on:

- Age of the youngest borrower
- Current interest rate
- The appraised home value or the FHA insurance limit, whichever is less

Financial Requirements:

- No income or credit qualifications
- No repayment as long as home serves as the primary residence
- You pay only the costs of appraisal and counseling (these fees may be financed)

Paying Off the Mortgage

The reverse mortgage is due when all owners leave or sell the home, or it passes to the heirs. Heirs may either pay the balance due and keep the home or sell the home and pay off the mortgage.

Repaying Your Loan

A HECM loan must be repaid in full when the owner dies or sells the home. The loan may also become due and payable if:

- You fail to pay property taxes, hazard insurance or violate other obligations.
- You permanently move to a new principal residence.

- You, or the last borrower, fail to live in the home for 12 months in a row — for example, if you were to stay in a nursing home for 12 months or more.

- You allow the property to deteriorate and do not make necessary repairs.

Who's a Good Fit for Reverse Mortgages

A reverse mortgage is a good fit for you if:

- You want to stay in your home for a long period of time

- You're *house rich* but *cash poor*.

- You're over 80, and need money for medical expenses or home care

- You're between the ages of 62 and 72, find your assets diminishing, need help to get by or just need to pay off your existing mortgage

- Your spouse requires senior care at home

As with any loan, borrowers must satisfy certain eligibility requirements. Borrowers must be at least 62 years of age. All homeowners must sign the loan papers. And most importantly, owners must occupy the home as a principal residence.

The following property types are eligible for reverse mortgage loans, and must meet all FHA property standards and flood requirements:

- Single family home or 1-4 unit home (with one unit occupied by the borrower)

- HUD-approved condominium or manufactured home

Mobile homes and co-op units are not eligible.

Who Reverse Mortgages Are Not For

- Seniors without long term care insurance who need to relocate to a senior care community

- Families that have owned the home for generations and want to continue to pass it on

- Married couples who do not have both names on the property title

- Married couples where one spouse is under the age of 62 and the younger lives in the home

- Seniors whose homes have very low property values

What is a *Jumbo* or *Proprietary* Reverse Mortgage?

Jumbo or *proprietary* reverse mortgages were structured and backed by private companies and designed for high value homes. These types of reverse mortgages are currently not available largely due to the prevailing credit crunch that is making loans harder to come by. Jumbo reverse mortgages are particularly risky at this time for several reasons:

- **Declining home values**: Since the home serves as collateral on a reverse mortgage loan, declining values makes this a risky loan option for lenders.

- **Lack of faith in banks:** The general perception about private banking institutions' solvency has made jumbo reverse mortgages highly unpopular unlike federally-backed HECM loans.

- **Limited secondary market**: Loans are often originated by one bank and then resold on a secondary market. Currently, Wall Street is not buying jumbo loans.

As home values have been declining and the credit crunch has impacted a bank's ability to resell mortgages, jumbo reverse mortgages have become too risky for most lenders to offer.

Myths About Reverse Mortgages

Myth #1: A reverse mortgage sells the home to the bank

False. Lenders are generally not in the business of owning homes -- they wish to make loans and earn interest. The homeowner keeps the title, and the lender adds a lien onto the title for the amount that is borrowed. In this way, the lender guarantees repayment.

Myth #2: Heirs will not inherit the home

False. The estate inherits the home as usual but there will be a lien on the title for the balance of the reverse mortgage. The balance equals proceeds received from the reverse mortgage, plus closing costs, fees and interest.

Myth #3: The homeowner could get forced out of the home

False. The HECM reverse mortgage was designed to allow seniors to live in their home for as long as they are able to. Because the homeowner *receives* payments from a reverse mortgage instead of making payments to a lender, the homeowner can never be evicted or foreclosed on for non-payment. As covered previously in this chapter, the borrower can default on the loan for other reasons.

Myth #4: Someone can outlive a reverse mortgage

False. The older you are, the more money you can receive (because of a lower life expectancy). As a general rule, if you selected the monthly payment option and outlive your life expectancy, the reverse mortgage lender must continue to make payments each month even if the total principal and accrued interest exceed your home's market value.

Myth #5: Social Security and Medicare will be affected

False. Government entitlement programs such as Social Security and Medicare are not affected by a reverse mortgage. However, need-based programs such as Medicaid *can* be affected. To remain eligible for Medicaid, the borrower must not make monthly reverse mortgage withdrawals that would exceed the Medicaid limits.

Myth #6: The homeowner pays taxes on reverse mortgage proceeds

False. The proceeds from a reverse mortgage are not considered income and therefore, are not taxable. Furthermore, the interest on a reverse mortgage is tax deductible when it is repaid in full.

Myth #7: There are large out-of-pocket expenses

False. Typically, the only out-of-pocket expenses are the cost of the counseling and the appraisal. If requested, these fees may also be financed.

Myth #8: A reverse mortgage is similar to a home equity loan

False. The only similarity between a reverse mortgage and a home equity loan is that both use the home's equity as collateral. There are several differences between the two, including:

- Any homeowner can apply for a home equity loan. Reverse mortgages are for seniors age 62 and up.

- A home equity loan must be repaid in monthly payments over 5 or 10 years. A reverse mortgage is not paid back until the homeowner moves out of the property or passes away.

- A home equity loan requires stable income and a solid credit score. A reverse mortgage does not consider income or credit score as factors.

- A home equity loan charges no closing costs but has a higher interest rate over the life of the loan. A reverse mortgage charges upfront closing costs, but may have a lower interest rate over the course of the loan.

Taxes, Estates, and Public Benefits

Reverse mortgages may have tax consequences, affect eligibility for federal and state programs, and have an impact on the estate and heirs.

According to the American Bar Association, "the IRS does not consider loan advances to be income." However, if you receive SSI, Medicaid, or other public benefits, loan advances are counted as "liquid assets" if you keep them in an account past the end of the calendar month in which you receive them. In this case, you could lose eligibility for these programs if your total liquid assets (e.g., savings and checking accounts) exceed program limits.

HECM counselors should discuss program eligibility requirements, financial implications and alternatives to obtaining a HECM. They should also discuss conditions for the mortgage becoming due and payable. Upon the completion of HECM counseling, you should be able to make an independent, informed decision as to whether this product will meet your needs. You can find an HECM counselor online at HUD's website: http://www.hud.gov/offices/hsg/sfh/hecm/hecmlist.cfm.

As mentioned previously, a reverse mortgage calculator will help you determine if you qualify. If you meet the eligibility criteria, you can complete a reverse mortgage application by contacting an FHA-approved lender. HUD has a list of approved vendors on their website: http://www.hud.gov/ll/code/llslcrit.cfm.

HECM Costs: A Rundown of Additional Fees & Expenses

As with any other type of loan, the HECM loan involves some additional costs, including an **origination fee**, **closing costs**, **mortgage insurance premium**, **interest** and **servicing fees**. These additional costs can be financed and paid using the proceeds from the loan.

The **origination fee** compensates the lender for processing your loan. A lender can charge a HECM origination fee up to $2,500 if your home is valued at less than $125,000. If your home is valued at more than $125,000 lenders can charge 2% of the first $200,000 of your home's value plus 1% of the amount over $200,000. HECM origination fees are capped at $6,000.

Third party **closing costs** can cover an appraisal, title search and insurance, surveys, inspections, recording fees, mortgage taxes, credit checks and other fees.

Mortgage insurance guarantees that you will receive expected loan advances and that you will not have to repay the loan for as long as you live in your home. The insurance also guarantees that, if you or your heirs sell your home to repay the loan, your total debt can never be greater than the value of your home.

The **mortgage insurance premium (MIP)** can be financed as part of your loan. You will be charged an upfront MIP at closing which will equal 2% of the lesser of your home's value or the FHA HECM mortgage limit for your area. You will also be charged a monthly MIP that equals 0.5% of the mortgage balance.

Lenders will charge a servicing fee throughout the life of the loan for such maintenance as sending account statements, disbursing loan proceeds, and tax and insurance notifications. Monthly servicing fees will not exceed $30 if the loan has an annually adjusting interest rate or $35 if the loan has a monthly adjusting interest rate. At loan origination, HECM lenders deduct the servicing fee from your available funds. Each month thereafter, the monthly servicing fee is added to your loan balance.

HECM borrowers can choose an adjustable interest rate or a fixed rate. An adjustable interest rate may be adjusted monthly or annually. Lenders may not adjust annually adjusted HECMs by more than 2 percentage points per year and not by more than 5 total percentage points over the life of the loan. FHA does not require interest rate caps on monthly-adjusted HECMs.

HECM Housing Counselor Lists

FHA funds housing counseling agencies throughout the country that can provide unbiased, accurate advice about reverse mortgages. To find a counselor near you, visit the FHA Housing Counseling Agency Listings at the Web site below, or call (800) 569-4287.

http://www.hud.gov/offices/hsg/sfh/hcc/hcs.cfm?filtersvc=hec&filtermultistate=yes

You may also contact a HECM counselor from FHA's National HECM Counseling Network, found at:

http://www.hud.gov/offices/hsg/sfh/hcc/hccprof18.cfm

Things to Look Out For

Here are some things you should consider when seeking a reverse mortgage agent:

- **Personal referrals**: Ask friends, neighbors, and colleagues you trust for referrals for a reputable agent.

- **Client referrals**: A competent and trustworthy agent should be more than willing to provide you with referrals from satisfied clients. Contact at least two or three of them to get honest feedback about the quality of service they received.

- **Make sure your agent is licensed.** The agent should be in good standing with your state's governing board. It makes sense to validate this using the license number and/or the license number of the broker if they are working underneath one.

- **Do they have a quota?** It is completely fair to ask potential agents if they're working on a monthly quota system. If so, they may not have your best interests at heart.

- **Seek an agent who works with financial planners:** It's a matter of common sense; providing yourself with a team of knowledgeable people is really smart!

- **Ask them if they're familiar with the** *National Aging in Place Council***'s Code of Conduct.**

- **Seek advice and support** from a trusted family member or friend.

- **Trust your gut:** A reverse mortgage loan is a big decision. If the agent ever makes you feel rushed or uncomfortable, keep looking.

Special Thanks

A special thanks goes out to Linda Lewis who graciously shared her wealth of knowledge on the subject of reverse mortgages. Linda resides in Orange County, California. Her contact information is below.

Linda Lewis
Reverse Mortgage Specialist
FutureSafe Financial Corporation
www.ReverseWithLinda.com
Phone: 949-278-4392 and 800-456-7542

Need a Provider in Your State?

Inside Elder Care maintains a list of reverse mortgage providers nationwide. For a list of reverse mortgage providers in your state, visit www.insideeldercare.com/reverse-mortgages.

Using Veterans' Pension Benefits

There are two types of cash benefits available for U.S. veterans: *compensation* and *pension*. *Compensation* is a benefit provided to veterans that have suffered a disability as a result of their military service. *Pension* benefits are more common — they are available to veterans with limited or no income that served during a war period. Pension benefits can help veterans and their surviving spouses to cover a large portion, if not all, of their medical and eldercare costs.

What are Veterans' Pension Benefits?

Veterans' pension benefits are available to veterans who served on active duty during a period of war or to the single surviving spouses of these veterans. About 33% of all seniors in the U.S. could qualify for up to $1,949 a month in additional income from the Department of Veterans Affairs (VA). This resource is a great way to fund elder care services at home provided that adequate documentation is provided to the VA.

Of approximately 35 million Americans age 65 and older, about 11.5 million are veterans who served during a period of war. To qualify for pension benefits, the veteran must:

- Have served 90 days of active duty, at least one day of which was during a wartime period (24 months if service was after 1980).[1]

- Have been discharged under conditions other than dishonorable.

---

1 The 90-day requirement can be split between different wars; it's sometimes been the case that veterans served in both World War II and the Korean Conflict.

- Be over 65 years of age *or* 100% disabled.

There is sometimes ambiguity about these criteria, but the most important thing to remember is that these benefits only apply to *wartime* vets.[2] Thus, there are millions of vets who didn't serve during a war that do not qualify for pension benefits.

If you're the widow or widower of a war-time veteran...

- You must have been married to the veteran at the time of the veteran's death.

- You must have been married to the veteran for at least 12 months, unless you had a child.

- You cannot have divorced the veteran (there are very limited exceptions).

- You cannot have remarried (there are some exceptions).

— Jim Swain, VA Accredited Attorney
Founder of the Academy of VA Pension Planners

At this point you'll have a good idea if the senior in question qualifies for veterans' long-term care assistance. If the basic criteria have been met, let's move on to a brief discussion of income and assets requirements for pension eligibility.

When it comes to income, the following requirements apply:

- Income must be less than the maximum pension for the classification after subtracting the un-reimbursed medical expenses of the veteran or the widow.

- All income from all sources of the veteran and any dependent must be counted.

- All social security benefits must also be counted, not just the taxable portion.

---

2 Despite the fact that they were never declared wars, vets that served in Vietnam and Korea both qualify as mandated by Congress. Veterans of the Gulf War, which began in 1990 and is still ongoing, qualify for the benefit. However, many soldiers who served in the Gulf war, including those who serve today in Afghanistan or Iraq, never served the required 24 months of consecutive service.

The following guidelines apply to the veteran's assets:

- The total amount of "countable assets" is limited to the amount that is reasonably expected to be utilized within the veteran or widow's lifetime.

- Countable assets do not include the residence, burial policies, small life insurance policies, personal property or auto.

- A single claimant is allowed approximately $50,000 of countable assets; a married couple is allowed up to $80,000.

- There is no rule that limits the claimant's exact amount of countable assets, but it is left to the discretion of the claims adjudicator. They will look at the current financial needs, assuming they receive the maximum pension benefit, and multiply these by the applicant's life expectancy.

- There is no rule against giving away assets to qualify.

- There is no penalty period for gifting away assets. See a knowledgeable attorney before gifting away assets to avoid income tax issues or Medicaid disqualification.

What Assistance is Available?

There are three levels of veterans' pension benefits: *basic pension, pension with Housebound Assistance* and *pension with Aid & Attendance.* Each classification has certain medical requirements, and in all cases, the veteran must be over the age of 65 or 100% disabled to qualify.

The **basic pension** is the lowest payment level. There are no eligibility requirements based on medical need.

The pension with **Housebound benefit** is for housebound veterans who are unable to drive and unable to leave home without assistance. The claimant does not necessarily need to be disabled to qualify for this classification of benefits.

The pension with **Aid and Assistance benefit** is for seniors who require assistance with at least three of their activities of daily living described in Chapter 3. This is the highest pension amount and is determined by the applicant's health.

All levels of the pension benefit have income and asset requirements. It is recommended that you apply even if in doubt about your ability to meet the requirements since the VA sometimes grants exceptions under special circumstances. Consult someone who has a thorough understanding of the VA Pension Program and can help you obtain all the benefits that you are entitled to.

Applying for Pension Benefits: Things to Remember

- The criteria regarding wartime service and marital status are unambiguous.

- The criteria regarding income and assets and medical conditions have more room for interpretation.

- The pension benefit is based on the health of the *claimant* — if the veteran is married, only he or she is the claimant; if the veteran is deceased, the surviving spouse is the claimant.

- Everything must be documented by the senior's physician. Talk with your doctor to make sure that his or her documentation of your condition accurately reflects your needs. For example, don't let your doctor get away with reporting, "He does normal activities for an 87-year old." This is too vague and will not ensure that the senior veteran receives all the benefits he is entitled to.

- In some cases, service-related disability payments (i.e., benefits received as a result of injury while on duty) may be available to the veteran and his or her family, but the veteran may only receive the higher of the two.

- You can apply for service-related disability *and* pension benefits simultaneously. If the disability is approved, the service-related disability benefits will be offset by the pension payments that have been received.

Don't Rely on the VA – Be sure to Consult an Expert

"We have often helped potential applicants receive the benefit even when they have been told by VA that they do not qualify," shared Jim Swain. "This third level of pension income is often used to pay costs of long term care such as home care, assisted living or nursing home care. That's because the nature of these expenditures allows potential applicants for the aid and attendance benefit to meet the special provisions of the income test."

How VA Pension Benefits Work

If the senior is *over* 65, they are presumed to be disabled and unemployable by Veterans Affairs. If they are under the age of 65, the burden of proof is heavier and requires the applicant's doctor to fully document the exact nature of their condition and abilities.

How to Assess Your Eligibility

The Department of Veterans Affairs uses "income for VA purposes" (IVAP) to determine eligibility. It is important to note that this figure actually refers to an *adjusted income,* not the gross annual income. You or your advisor can determine your IVAP by subtracting any unreimbursed, recurring medical expenses from the gross annual income. Countable medical expenses refer to any kind of in-home care, co-pays, or medical supplies that assist a senior with their ADLs.[3]

IVAP limits are as follows:

- If married, yearly income cannot exceed $23,388

- If single, yearly income cannot exceed $19,728

- If widowed, yearly income cannot exceed $12,672

Gross Income – countable medical expenses = IVAP

---

[3] Prescription drug expenses are not eligible medical expenses because they are not consistent expenses.

For example, a veteran that has a monthly income of $2,400, and in-home care and additional medical expenses of $2,000 per month, would have an IVAP of $400 per month. If they qualify for a pension with Aid and Attendance, then they would be entitled to receive the difference between the maximum pension and their IVAP, which in this case, equals a monthly pension of $1,549 (i.e., $1,949 maximum pension - $400 IVAP = $1,549 monthly pension).

How is Net Worth a Factor in Determining Eligibility?

While Medicaid is quite specific about defining allowable net worth, VA simply states that the veteran is "not allowed to have more net worth than is reasonably expected to be utilized in their lifetime." The Department of Veterans Affairs takes a snapshot of net worth, income, and expense on a case-by-case basis to help determine eligibility.

For example, consider an 86-year-old veteran with a life expectancy of three years. VA regards only his life expectancy and not his health or medical records.[4] Taking into account income, VA pension, and medical expenses, he has a shortfall of $1,000 per month. Using a very simple equation, VA multiplies that $1,000 monthly shortfall by his life expectancy of 36 months to determine that $36,000 is his maximum need.

This formula, of course, is far too conservative — it doesn't take into account basic living expenses or inflation let alone other recurring costs like credit card or mortgage payments.

Much like Medicaid estate planners, VA pension planners try to restructure assets so that the veteran can qualify for the highest benefits. The difference is that the rules are very clear with Medicaid — a married couple can keep up to $104,600 in countable assets. VA benefits, however, are designed for veterans with limited income.

The strategy of many planners is to try to figure how much money the veteran can keep. Instead, it's smarter to plan differently, by focusing on how *little* the veteran is allowed to keep. After all, they may be

---

4 In August of 2009, the Center for Disease Control issued a press release: "U.S. life expectancy reached nearly 78 years (77.9). The report, "Deaths: Preliminary Data for 2007," was issued today by CDC's National Center for Health Statistics. The data are based on nearly 90 percent of death certificates in the United States. The 2007 increase in life expectancy – up from 77.7 in 2006 -- represents a continuation of a trend. Over a decade, life expectancy has increased 1.4 years from 76.5 years in 1997 to 77.9 in 2007. (http://www.cdc.gov/media/pressrel/2009/r090819.htm)

electing to apply for Medicaid benefits sometime in the future. With the 5-year look back rule, they will be penalized with a significant delay.

Currently the VA has no look-back period, meaning a veteran can give away their assets and apply for VA benefits the very next day in order to qualify. It's *how* the Veteran gives away the money that counts.[5]

Consider this example: In some states, an applicant could create a Special Needs Trust and thus qualify for Medicaid. Upon his or her death, Medicaid could recover their expenses from the trust. With the VA, if the applicant has any control over the trust, the agency will count the whole thing in determining net worth. Therefore, the trust must be owned by the veteran's children.

Who's a Good Fit for Veterans' Benefits?

Fundamentally, if you or your loved one is a veteran who meets the standards of service, then speak with a qualified VA Accredited Attorney to see what benefits they are entitled to. As described above, an attorney can help you review income and assets and strategize the best way to restructure assets for the highest possible benefits.

Keep in mind that most pension applications are reviewed on a case-by-case basis, so it doesn't hurt to apply if you meet the most basic criteria of military service.

What to Look For in a VA Pension Planner

Only VA employees, trained veterans' service officers, and VA accredited attorneys are able to assist you with the VA pension benefits application. Further, no one can charge you for their assistance with the application. An attorney can *only* charge for adjunct activities such as trusts, wills, financial reviews, powers of attorney and/or income tax analysis. That said, keep the following in mind when seeking out a VA pension planner:

- Make sure the planner has at least 2 years experience in VA pension planning, a background in estate planning and extensive knowledge of Medicaid, tax law, and elder law.

- Ask the planner where he or she was trained.

---

5 Unlike Medicaid, the VA has no regulatory legislation. It is governed only by General Counsel Opinions which are over 14 years old.

- Ask the planner for references — and follow through on contacting those references.

- Be wary of a planner who is pushing an annuity. Annuities aren't necessarily bad, but it's important to feel comfortable that a planner is truly assessing what will work best for you.

- As with anyone you choose to hire for your eldercare, listen to your gut. An ideal VA planner is a compassionate listener and will take the time to work through the details of your story.

- Though it is wise to seek advice, take ownership of the process. Don't be intimidated by the status of "attorney." Ask questions about their educational background, their experience and trust your intuition.

You can start your search for a VA accredited attorney or agent here: http://vabenefits.vba.va.gov/vonapp/other_partners.asp.

Things to Watch Out For

Especially if you do have assets to declare, keep in mind the following:

- Naming more than one owner on an account can reduce the declarable assets, but guardianship courts can order the other parties to remove their names from the accounts. This could disqualify the applicant for VA benefits and require them to repay past benefit payments.

- Moving IRAs can be challenging. They're both an asset and an income stream and can pose tax liabilities. It helps to consult an attorney who will assess the tax-liability of all your assets.

- Is the senior a beneficiary of anyone? If someone is planning to leave them money, consider having them change their will to eliminate disqualification of the senior for VA or Medicaid benefits.

- Though a home is not a countable asset, a veteran could be disqualified from receiving benefits — and be required to pay back past benefits — if they sell the house. If the senior is planning to sell, discuss it early on with your pension planner.[6]

Can a Veteran Receive Both VA Benefits and Medicaid?

If a single veteran goes on Medicaid they will give up all their income and they'll give up most of their VA pension. They can only keep a state-mandated amount of their income plus $90 per month in pension benefits. It is more complex for married couples, and most cases are reviewed on an individual basis. Consult a VA pension planner.

Special Thanks

A special thanks goes to Jim Swain, a VA-accredited attorney and a Navy veteran who teaches VA Pension Planning techniques to estate and elder law attorneys. Jim is the founder of the Academy of VA Pension Planners that certifies VA Planners. It is a valuable clearinghouse of information for veterans and their families. You can learn more about Jim or the AVAPP by visiting his website, http://www.avapp.org, or contacting him directly.

James B. "Jim" Swain
Academy of VA Pension Planners
515 E. Crossville Road, Suite 100
Roswell, GA. 30075
Phone: 888-928-2779
Fax: 770-587-0050
jim@avapp.org

Need a Provider in Your State?

Inside Elder Care maintains a list of VA Pension benefit specialists nationwide. For a list of VA Pension benefit specialists in your state, visit www.insideeldercare.com/VA-Benefit.

---

6 It is commonly advised that the veteran decline the benefits, sell the house, gift the money and then reapply for VA benefits once their income and assets are realigned with VA requirements. Capital gains from the sale of the house are taxable, so the senior could find themselves in a deep financial hole. As always, seek the advice from an accredited VA or tax attorney.

FIVE

LIFE SETTLEMENTS

Many seniors purchased life insurance policies when they were younger — most likely when they got married, had children or bought a home. They've made payments on the policy but now find that their needs have changed. A life settlement is a transaction wherein a policyholder sells his or her life insurance policy to an institutional investor.

Typically, these investors pay much more for insurance policies than their cash "surrender" values. Because most life insurance values are guaranteed and disconnected from the economy, there is no fluctuation, as is the case, with real estate and stocks. And, almost every type of life insurance contract can be used for a life settlement.

The proceeds from the settlement can be used to pay for in-home care, assisted living or nursing home care that's needed now.

Glossary of Terms

Face Value: The face value of a life insurance policy is the death benefit. In the case of so-called "double indemnity" life insurance policies, the beneficiary receives double the face value in case of accidental death.

Cash Surrender Value: The amount available in cash upon cancellation of an insurance policy, usually a whole life policy, before it becomes payable upon death or maturity. This is also called cash value or surrender value.

How it Works

A life settlement is an alternative way for seniors to generate cash for immediate needs by selling their life insurance policy and receiving a lump sum payment in return. This is not a loan, which means the funds are unrestricted and require no repayment.

If your life insurance policy has a cash surrender value, you can cash in your policy with your insurer at any time during the policy and receive that amount. A life settlement, however, can yield a much larger return than a surrender value. An investor *buys* your insurance policy, therefore, becoming the beneficiary. Upon your death, the investor will receive the death benefit.

The gains from a life settlement may be tax deductible if used to pay for in-home care, assisted living or skilled nursing care. Naturally, you should talk with a qualified tax accountant to learn if deductibility applies to your situation.

Almost any type of life insurance may be eligible for a life settlement transaction, including term, universal life, whole life, survivorship and key-man policies.

Types of Life Insurance

Term insurance, the simplest type of insurance, provides coverage for only a specified period. If you die during that term, your beneficiary receives the value of the policy. There is no investment component, and therefore, it has no cash surrender value.

Whole Life insurance covers your *whole life* rather than just a specified period. Premiums remain level throughout the life of the policy, and the company invests at least a portion of your premiums. Some firms share investment proceeds with policyholders in the form of a dividend. Many companies will offer a relatively low guaranteed rate of return, but in reality pay at a rate greater than the guarantee.

Universal Life insurance combines term or whole life insurance with an investment vehicle. The policyholder decides on a premium payment, and funds that exceed the cost of insurance go into a cash-value account—the proceeds from which can be used against premiums or allowed to grow. The insurance company chooses the investment vehicle which are typically bonds and mortgages. Sometimes called Type I or Type A policies, the cash account goes toward the death benefit. A second variety, sometimes called Type II or Type B, allows the beneficiary to receive the face value of the policy plus all or most of the cash account. A variation of a universal policy, often called universal variable life, allows policyholders to choose investment vehicles.

Key Man insurance (also known as Key Person or Business Life) is an insurance policy that covers a company's executive, founder or owner. In the event of the sudden loss of that person, the company's operations would be significantly injured. The company is the beneficiary of the plan and therefore pays the insurance policy premiums. The death benefit essentially buys the company time to recruit a replacement or to implement other strategies to save the business.

Survivorship Life insurance (also known as Joint and Survivor insurance or Second-to-Die Life insurance) is a policy that insures the lives of two people, typically a married couple. The death benefit is not paid to the beneficiary until the death of the second insured. This type of policy is generally available as either a whole or universal life policies, and it is a more affordable alternative to buying separate policies within a family.

If your life insurance policy has a cash value, the amount you receive should be greater than the cash surrender value. Contact your insurance company to find out the cash surrender value of your policy.

A life settlement broker will determine their offer for your policy based on the following:

- The age and medical condition of the insured
- Type of life insurance policy (e.g., universal life, whole life, term)
- The amount of the death benefit
- The rating of the issuing insurance company
- The amount of premiums necessary to keep the policy in force
- The amount of compensation the life settlement broker will receive

I recommend that you compare offers from several life settlement companies before selling your policy. Since you will be providing personal information to obtain quotes, be sure the companies you deal with have procedures in place to protect the confidentiality of your information.

The ownership rights and obligations are transferred to a new owner, and a new beneficiary will receive the proceeds upon the death of the insured. This is an important decision that may have significant financial consequences for you and your family members. As such, you may want to include your family as part of your decision-making process before making any major changes to your life insurance policy.

Work closely with a qualified advisor throughout the **8 steps of a life settlement transaction:**

1. Consult with an advisor before deciding to sell the policy.

2. Along with your advisor, decide whether to work with broker or to go directly to providers.

3. Submit your policy for valuation. At this point, investors will ask for sensitive information, such as medical history, to make an informed offer.

4. If your policy meets the criteria for a life settlement, providers will send offers directly or through a broker.

5. Review all offers and accept the optimum bid.

6. Complete the provider's closing package, and return essential documents.

7. The provider places cash payment in escrow and submits change of ownership forms to the insurance carrier.

8. Paperwork is verified and funds are transferred to the policy seller in one lump payment.

The process usually takes between 90 and 110 days — a relatively short turnaround time for a significant eldercare solution.

Why Consider a Life Settlement?

There are many reasons to choose life settlement, including funding eldercare expenses. Some reasons people settle their life insurance assets include:

- Reduce or eliminate life insurance premium payments
- Enable or maintain a more comfortable lifestyle in retirement
- Fund new annuities, life insurance, long-term care or investments
- Fund the purchase of a survivorship policy
- Settle personal or business debts
- Bestow cash gifts to family members or charities
- Boost cash flow by eliminating future premiums
- Activate income from an inactive asset
- Generate more cash than surrendering the policy or letting it lapse

— Rick Gardner, www.lifestylesettlements.com

Who's a Good Fit for Life Settlements?

The insured should be over the age of 60, and the typical client is over the age of 74. In a life settlement transaction, age as a criterion is flexible because age is less important than *life expectancy*. Typically, life settlement clients have a life expectancy of less than 12 years which is determined by a third-party review of medical records. Naturally, there can be variances in this estimation generating different offers from different investors. This is where a good broker works the hardest — by negotiating with the funding sources.

Life settlement is best suited to people who have an insurance policy with a face value over $100,000. The policy must have been active for more than two years, have a low cash surrender value and the yearly premiums should be less than 8% of the face value.

Who isn't a Good Candidate for Life Settlement?

Life settlement may not be suitable for your eldercare funding if the expected lifespan of the insured is longer than 12 years. The same is true for policyholders with higher cash surrender values.

A life settlement is also not ideal for someone who has dependents who will rely on the policy proceeds (for long term care, for instance) after the policyholder's death. If a life settlement would leave a spouse or dependent without any life insurance coverage or the ability to buy new insurance, then it may well be the wrong choice.

Lastly, if a person does not qualify to purchase new insurance coverage due to a medical condition, then it may not be suitable to pursue a life settlement.

There is a special transaction available for individuals who have a life expectancy of less than 36 months called **viatical settlement**.

Viatical Settlements

Like a life settlement, a *viatical settlement* is the sale of a life insurance policy before the policy matures. Generally, viatical settlements are for insured individuals with a shorter life expectancy. This can be a practical way to pay extremely high health insurance costs faced by severely, terminally ill people. The proceeds from a viatical settlement are not taxable.

Viatical settlements became prevalent in the United States in the late 1980s. Viatical settlements offered a way to extract value from the policy while the policyholder was still alive. Later, the frequency of unscrupulous private lenders led to a decline in viatical settlements and increased government regulation.

Three Examples

To better understand how a life settlement could benefit a senior facing elder care costs, let's consider three hypothetical scenarios.

First consider a married couple that holds a **survivorship policy**; the husband is 87 years old and his wife, a year younger. The face value of the policy is $600,000, but only has a cash value of $1,500 — the amount of money he would receive in surrendering the policy to the insurance company. A life settlement could offer him $81,000.

The second scenario involves a 78-year old man, who holds a **key person universal life policy**. As the insured, he had the right to assume ownership of the policy but no longer needed coverage. The policy has a $500,000 face value, and a cash surrender value of

$35,000. A life settlement could bring him $85,768 – well over 200% of the surrender value.

Lastly, consider an 88-year old man with a universal life policy. The face value was $325,000, and the cash value a significant $44,000. But, through life settlement, the offer made to the policy owner could be as much as $90,021 – again over 200% of the cash surrender value.

What to Look Out For

As with the other funding options described in this book, a life settlement is an important decision, and it's always recommended to consult a tax advisor and a legal advisor—not your general purpose financial advisor. When considering a life settlement, keep in mind the following:

- Life settlement proceeds may be taxable. You should consult your tax advisor about this.

- Consult your legal advisor before entering into a life settlement contract.

- Seek a broker that has connections with reputable, large institutional investors as opposed to private lenders or small institutions.

- Deal with a broker who has access to all the capital market buyers.

- Make sure the broker has Errors and Omissions insurance.

- Ask for proof of license if your state is regulated. (Some states, including California and New York, have no regulatory stipulations.)

- Turn to the *Federal Trade Commission* to see if there are any complaints about the broker.

- Ask the broker for references and follow through on those references.

- Ask your broker to see the bid history—you deserve a transparent transaction.

- Only work with a broker who is willing to disclose his or her commission.

- Work with a broker who has at least 5 years experience with life settlements.

- Only deal with brokers who are willing to have a face-to-face personal interview with you and your financial advisor or eldercare attorney.

How Does a Life Settlement Compare to a Reverse Mortgage?

Both a life settlement and a reverse mortgage access cash from an existing asset. How are they different?

As discussed in Chapter 3, a reverse mortgage is a loan that will accrue interest and incur fees. It must be paid back once the homeowner no longer occupies the home as their primary residence. The size of a reverse mortgage loan is determined by the borrower's age, the interest rate and the home's value. The older the borrower, the larger the percentage of the home's value that can be borrowed. The Federal Housing Administration, which is part of HUD, collects an insurance premium (2% on average) from all borrowers as part of the financing agreement.

Unlike a reverse mortgage loan, a life settlement is the *sale* of personal property. The proceeds from the sale are unrestricted, and there are no payback requirements. There is no cap as to how much money can be generated from a life settlement—nor are there interest fees, guarantees, or liens. Also unlike reverse mortgages, life settlements have no income or asset requirements, and the price for a policy is determined in the open market through a competitive bidding process. As mentioned previously, the proceeds from a life settlement can be taxable, and each case needs to be assessed individually by a certified tax advisor. Typically, the taxable proceeds are based on the difference between the cost basis of a policy (the money paid in) and the cash "surrender" value and the final settlement amount received by the policy holder.

Can Life Settlements Impact Eligibility for Social Assistance Programs

Yes. Funds derived from a life settlement may affect eligibility for needs-based public assistance programs such as Medicaid, aid to families with dependent children, supplementary social security income and AIDS drug assistance programs. It is important to note that life insurance is characterized as an "unprotected" asset for Medicaid applicants and the value of a policy typically exceeding $2,000 will count against the applicant's minimum allowable asset level.

Every state's Medicaid requirements vary, and I strongly recommend that a policy owner consult with the appropriate social services agency or a financial advisor concerning how ownership of a life insurance policy and a subsequent life settlement could affect your eligibility and that of your spouse or dependents.

Pre-Qualification Worksheet

Use this worksheet as a tool to help you determine if life settlement is a viable option for funding your eldercare.

Part A requires score of 5 or higher. Total A & B of 15 points or greater — considered a prime candidate for Life Settlement

	Add Points	Part A-Insured	
1 pt		Male 75 or younger	Female 77 or younger
2 pts		Male 76-80	Female 78-82
3 pts		Male 81-83	Female 83-85
4 pts		Male 84 or older	Female 86 or older
1 pt		In good health	
2 pts		Minor health problems	
3 pts		Significant health change since policy issue	
4 pts		Serious health problems	
		Part B-The Policy	
1 pt		Whole Life	
2 pts		Survivorship	
3 pts		Convertible Term	

4 pts		Universal or Joint Survivorship with 1 deceased
1 pt		Cash or loan value exceeds 30% of death benefit
2 pts		Cash or loan value 20%-29% of death benefit
3 pts		Cash or loan value 10%-19% of death benefit
4 pts		Cash or loan value less than 10% of death benefit
1 pt		Premium exceeds 7% of death benefit
2 pts		Premium 5%-7% of death benefit
3 pts		Premium 3%-5% of death benefit
4 pts		Premium 3% or less than death benefit
Total Score		

Special Thanks

Special thanks to Rick Gardner, of *LifeStyle Settlements, Inc.*, who provided a great deal of insight into life settlements. Rick is located in Orange County, California and can be reached below.

Rick Gardner
LifeStyle Settlements, Inc.
30448 Rancho Viejo Rd. Suite 250
San Juan Capistrano, CA 92675
(800)-493-2056 Ext. 267
Phone: 949-272-2267
rgardner@lifestylesettlements.com

Need a Provider in Your State?

Inside Elder Care maintains a list of life settlement providers nationwide. For a list of life settlement providers in your state, visit www.insideeldercare.com/life-settlements

SENIOR LIVING LINES OF CREDIT

What is a Senior Living Line of Credit?

A senior living line of credit allows people to "buy some time" and liquidate assets at the best possible return in order to pay for a senior's housing and care needs.

Sometimes eldercare is an urgent need, and other funding resources — such as proceeds from the sale of a home, stocks and bonds, and pension or veteran benefits — are not immediately available. This unsecured line of credit is typically up to $50,000. A senior living line of credit can give your family some breathing room and time. It can enable the senior to get settled in his or her new assisted living community, and it can give you the time necessary to evaluate longer-term financial plans to fund the care your loved one needs.

How it Works

Some companies, such as *Elderlife Financial Services*, require that a family select a community from their network of approved facilities in order to qualify. By using a network of communities, consumers can be reasonably assured that every community is screened to ensure a high standard of care.[1] Elderlife's assisted living locator tool is a great place to start: http://www.elderlifefinancial.com/locator/assisted_living_locator_home.aspx.

Visit multiple communities before deciding which community is right for your senior and your family. Speak with administrators to learn about upfront fees and monthly housing and care costs. Calculate the

---

1 Currently Elderlife Financial Services boasts a network of 2,500 eldercare facilities, and expect to grow to 3,100 member facilities by 2011.

senior's monthly income (e.g., from pension or social security) and assets available for liquidation.

A financial counseling session with an advisor will help a family to determine the line of credit they may need. The senior applies for this line of credit as holder of the assets, but typically the children or other family members are also named on the loan.

Six Steps to a Senior Living Line of Credit

1. Determine the monthly cost of care at your chosen community.

2. Determine any additional monthly costs related to eldercare.

3. Determine any personal monthly costs not related to eldercare.

4. Determine the amount of financing the family has been approved for.

5. Determine how much your elder can afford to pay out-of-pocket each month.

6. Determine how much *you* can contribute to your elder's care cost needs each month.

What Assets Can Be Considered?

When determining sources of income for your senior, it's important to distinguish *between direct cash flow sources and illiquid assets*. Direct cash flow sources include such things as social security, pensions, long term care insurance policies and savings accounts.

Illiquid assets include such things as houses and life insurance policies. In addition to simply determining their value, you should also consider to what degree you plan to use them to fund eldercare needs and how long it may take to liquidate the assets.

Senior Living Line of Credit Worksheet

Use this worksheet to help determine if a senior living line of credit is a good fit for your family.

		Example
Monthly senior community cost	_____	$3,500
Additional monthly costs	_____	$500
Total monthly costs	_____	$4,000
Less out-of-pocket contributions from the senior	_____	$1,000
Monthly gap supplemented by family	_____	$3,000
Multiplied by number of months you estimate are needed to sell the home or supplement a monthly shortfall on behalf of a loved one?	_____	8
Subtotal of estimated credit line amount needed	_____	$24,000
Plus one-time move-in or security deposit	_____	$ 3,000
Total senior living line of credit amount needed	_____	$27,000

This worksheet was provided by Elias Papasavvas of Elderlife Financial Services.

When determining costs, be aware of the differences between changing and unchanging costs. *Unchanging* costs are predictable, and will include the community's monthly rent and other community fees for things like food, transportation and laundry. *Changing* costs vary month-to-month and include things such as increased assistance with daily living activities, medication, clothing and doctor visits.

While the senior is on the line of credit, the adult children or other responsible parties typically need to guarantee the line. Although several kids can be on the loan, I recommend assigning a loan leader who is responsible for gathering the individual payments from your family and issuing one check to the creditor.

A Senior Living Credit Line is

- Structured to serve a senior and his or her family in an assisted living or senior living situation

- Unsecured

- Generally makes up to $50,000 available at a time

- Allows you to use only what you need, as you need it

- Makes it easy for attorneys, accountants, judges, to verify that funds were used for your loved one's assisted living housing and care

- Monitored, in that the monthly rent is sent directly to the community on your family's behalf

Most families use senior lines of credit for one to eighteen months, or until a liquidating event takes place. Other families with fewer or no assets simply make payments on the loan and make a balloon payment at the end.

The payment is usually $7 -$12 per $1,000 borrowed, and you only pay interest on the actual amount borrowed not on the total line of credit. As with any loan, it is important to consider how you plan to repay the funds. Will the line be repaid after the senior's assets are liquidated? Or will family members collectively pay it back over time in small monthly payments?

Either way can work; what matters is what your family *wants* to do. By placing the senior on the line of credit, the loan documents should make it clear that the loan is solely for their housing and care. By setting up the loan documents in this way, it should make it easier to demonstrate to an estate trustee that the loan was your parent's obligation that must be satisfied before any estate is available per the will.

Why Not a Home Equity Line of Credit?

An equity line of credit on the senior's home is another option, but it is difficult to ensure that all the proceeds from the loan are funding long-term care expenses. Since a senior line of credit requires thorough documentation about the senior's eldercare needs, you and your family can avoid potential conflict over how the proceeds should be used, and be assured that your senior will have the funding to receive the resources and care they deserve.

Who is a Good Fit for a Senior Living Line of Credit?

A senior living line of credit is *only* for seniors who are moving into an assisted living, senior living or retirement community. Payments are sent directly to the care community, not by family members, thereby ensuring integrity on everyone's part.

Families use this when they need *time* and *flexibility* while waiting for access of other resources, such as the proceeds from a home sale or veterans' benefits. Many families may not need a month-to-month solution but simply need money to cover large, upfront costs, such as, first months' rent or move-in fees.

Who is Not a Good Fit for a Senior Living Line of Credit?

A senior living line of credit is not for seniors without a support system such as family, trusted financial planners or an eldercare attorney. Further, it is difficult to get approved as a single senior because it's likely that his or her income is insufficient to make payments. Seniors without family are urged to enlist a professional advisor to go over the paperwork.

Questions to Ask a Loan Broker

When seeking out a senior living line of credit provider, there are some big issues to consider. For instance, do they offer a dedicated senior living 'product,' or is their funding solution adapted from their current loan packages? Is there integrity of payment? In other words, does the lender send monthly checks directly to the eldercare facility? There are other questions too which should be asked to protect you and your senior from high interest rates or unscrupulous lenders:

- Are there penalties for pre payment?

- What happens if your payment is a day late? Does your interest rate go up?

- How much is the up-front fee?[2]

- Are funds sent directly to the assisted living community, so that you can ensure they are used for their intended purpose?

- Do they wire/electronically transfer the funds, or is a paper check 'cut' and mailed? I recommend you do business with a lender who electronically transfers funds since a check can get lost or tampered with.

- Will the loan amount solve your short-term needs?

- Is this line of credit, or is it a loan?

- Is the application short and easy to complete?

- How long does it take to get a decision?

- How long do you have to pay it back? Is that enough time for your family?

- Are monthly payments affordable and reasonable?

- What is the interest rate?

- Are there any penalty rates?

- Do the documents make it easy for you to segment the obligation in the event you want to get reimbursed by the senior's estate or when the home or other assets are sold?

- Can several members of the family take part in the application and be jointly liable?

- Does the lender have a relationship with the senior living community, so that in the event something goes wrong, you can get some some help?

- Will the lender help you with getting the application and funding done quickly?

- Do you get a good feeling that the lender understands what you are going through?

---

2 The origination and support fee generally ranges from 4-8%. Remember that since most senior living lines of credit are short-term loans, the bank doesn't make much money. If the lender isn't forthcoming about their upfront fees, don't do business with them.

- Is there adequate staff to answer questions or resolve issues in a timely way?

A senior living line of credit may be the most ideal short-term solution for your family's eldercare funding needs. But consider the implications and make sure that all family members understand them too. Your lender should give you and your family time to deliberate and reflect over this decision – and if they don't, go somewhere else.

Special Thanks

Special thanks to Elderlife Financial Services founder Elias Papasavvas for his expert contributions in this chapter. If a senior living line of credit seems to be a good solution for your family, I recommend you consider Elderlife Financial Services.

Elias Papasavvas
Founder and CEO
Elderlife Financial Services
http://www.elderlifefinancial.com
1054 31st Street NW
Suite 340
Washington D.C., 20007
Phone: 1-888-228-4500

SEVEN

MEDICAID ESTATE PLANNING

It's easy to get Medicare and Medicaid confused. What's the difference?

Medicare is a federally-funded entitlement program for retirees over the age of 65 who paid into the Social Security system for at least 10 quarters. The Social Security Act of 1965 was passed by Congress and signed by President Lyndon B. Johnson as amendments to the original Social Security legislation. In fact, at the bill-signing ceremony, President Johnson enrolled former President Harry S. Truman as the first Medicare beneficiary and presented him with the first Medicare card.[1]

Medicaid, on the other hand, is the health program for individuals and families with *low incomes* and *negligible resources*. It is a means-tested program that is jointly funded by the states and federal government and is managed by the states.[2] Medicaid serves certain eligible U.S. citizens and resident aliens including low-income adults and their children and people with certain disabilities. Medicaid is the largest source of funding for medical and health-related services for people with limited income in the United States.

What is Medicaid Estate Planning?

Medicaid estate planning is an approach to satisfying financial eligibility requirements for Medicaid which covers some types of long-term care. An individual's assets are sheltered to the extent of voluntarily becoming "impoverished" to meet eligibility criteria. It is basically a legal way to restructure assets so that an individual can qualify for Medicaid long-term care assistance.

---

1 http://www.ssa.gov/history/lbjsm.html
2 http://www.cms.hhs.gov/MedicaidGenInfo/

How Medicaid Estate Planning Works

The average span of nursing home care is 30 months, and the average monthly cost is $7,000. Based on those averages, a family could spend $210,000 to provide their senior loved one with the care they need.

It was once true that people would be forced to take drastic measures to qualify for Medicaid: they'd divorce their life-long spouse, spend all their money, sell their house, even give their money away to family, friends or a charity, just so they could be declared indigent.

But that changed in 1986 when Congress lightened the burden with new legislation. Further changes came along in 2005 with the Deficit Reduction Act.

Medicaid for nursing home care is funded under a broad ring of social programs known as welfare. To be eligible for this, you must be declared impoverished under specific guidelines. Each state operates its own Medicaid system conforming to the federal guidelines, but there are shades of differences from one state to another.

Every individual or family's circumstances are assessed on a case-by-case basis. Though there are differences between how each state treats Medicaid cases, there are several common factors that are taken into consideration:

- Marital status

- Home ownership

- Pension benefits or social security income

- Assets such as real estate, stocks and bonds, mineral interests, annuities and IRAs

- The existence of appropriately drafted legal documents such as a will, power of attorney, living wills, trusts or other similar estate and disability planning documents

- Mental competency — to change those documents and release assets

- The extent of family support

- Urgency of required care

Based on these factors, there are ways to restructure existing assets in order to qualify for Medicaid assistance:

- Convert the assets that Medicaid considers *countable* to those they consider exempt or inaccessible.

- Convert an asset into an income stream.

- Transfer assets to other persons whether in the family or outside the family.

- Exercise the provisions which allow a client to expand the amount of protected assets beyond the statutory limits. This is called *resource expansion*.

NOTE: Do not implement any strategy *without the input of an experienced attorney who understands Medicaid rules and regulations.*

What are Countable Resources?

Countable resources are assets which could prevent you from receiving Medicaid long-term care assistance. A financial planner experienced with aging issues can help you idenify which assets can be converted or transferred to enable you to qualify for Medicaid benefits.

- Checking Accounts

- Savings Accounts

- Certificates of Deposit

- Money Market Accounts

- Stocks

- Bonds • U.S. Savings Bonds

- Mutual Funds

- IRAs, 401k and 403b plans

- Annuities (some)

- Life Insurance with cash value (some)

- Land / Lots / Houses (other than personal residence)

- Oil, Gas and Mineral interests

~ Martin R. Sabel, www.mreldercareonline.com

Common Thinking

Most people initially consider giving away their assets, but this can be more complicated than it sounds. Transferring assets for the purpose of applying for Medicaid will likely cause a delay in benefits. This delay is based on a formula. The amount transferred is divided by the published monthly cost of nursing home care in that state to equal how many months the benefits will be delayed:

$$\underline{\textbf{Amount transferred}} = \textbf{Months delayed}$$
$$\textbf{Monthly cost of nursinghome care}$$

For example, a $100,000 transfer divided by the average cost of nursing home care in that state of $5,000 per month equals a *20 month delay*. During this delay, nursing home expenses must be paid for out-of-pocket.

Good record-keeping is essential if you decide to gift your money. Prior to the Deficit Reduction Act, the attachment point was the date when you made the gift. After 2006, it's the date of application to Medicaid. Furthermore, Medicaid has a 5-year look-back at your financial transactions. Thus, keep these things in mind:

- Document any transfers that are made

- Keep a record and receipts showing amounts of any transferred funds spent on the patient's care

- If transfers were made for a purpose other than Medicaid qualification, you must either document that the patient was healthy at the time of transfer, or that the transfer was part of an established pattern (such as gifts or routine charitable donations)

- Most importantly, *do not apply until you know you're eligible*. The way to verify this is with the aid of a competent eldercare law attorney.

Don't Fall for the Annuity Solution

Seniors are often advised by their insurance agent or financial planner to convert existing assets into an annuity which makes immediate distributions.

Annuities are not the panacea that some make them out to be. The rules have changed, so it is important to work with someone who knows the Medicaid rules in your state and is affiliated with an Elder Law attorney.

Prior to 2006, there was a lot more freedom and flexibility in using annuities. The big concern now is that the state must be made the first beneficiary of the annuity contract. For married people, this poses an interesting danger.

Consider this scenario: A married couple must reduce their $100,000 in assets to $50,000 to qualify. They are advised to buy a $50,000 annuity to do so. It is designed to pay out over the life expectancy of the wife in this case 12 years. If she dies sooner, the monthly stipend that was used to pay for the husband's nursing care is paid to the state. Their children lose out on their inheritance.

There is a solution, but chances are, neither the couple nor their financial advisor realize it—pay out over a shorter period.

For a single person, annuities provide a way to transfer part of his or her assets out while ensuring they have sufficient income to cover nursing care costs during the penalty period. You can actually structure the annuity payout for as long as the penalty occurs and still protect assets.

Five things that will not necessarily prevent eligibility for the single person:

- Home
- 1 car
- Pre-paid burials
- Pre-paid funerals
- $2,000 in total assets

Don't Go It Alone

Only a qualified expert will know the ins and outs of each state. Most of us are overwhelmed when bombarded with legal or bureaucratic jargon, so leave it to the professionals – it's well worth the expense.

A married couple's income can be the greater amount between the monthly income of the non-institutionalized spouse or $2,739. In other words, it is possible for the wife to earn and keep $3,000 a month working outside the home while her husband's $1,500 in benefits can fund his care in a nursing home.

Let's consider a converse scenario. Suppose the wife earns only $500 a month, and her husband earns $1,500 a month in benefits. She may still keep all of the income because it's under the $2,739 limit.

Income for a single person cannot exceed $2,022 per month.

If your income is greater than this, an elder law attorney can work with you to come to a solution. If your income is $6,000 a month, it may not be worth applying for Medicaid at all. Still, it is always advisable to consult with an expert—you never know.

In most situations, the community spouse (the one living at home) can keep half of the countable resources up to a maximum of $109,560. Good estate planning may expand that, but it depends on your circumstances.

Who is a Good Fit for Medicaid Estate Planning?

As mentioned earlier, Medicaid rules and regulations vary from state to state but fall within these guidelines. Medicaid estate planning is best for:

- People with modest income (less than $3,000/month) with countable assets less than $600,000

- Anyone who has given assets away within the last five years

- Anyone with a strong family support system

- Anyone who owns a home

Who Is Not a Good Fit for Medicaid Estate Planning?

Medicaid Estate Planning does not work for seniors who want to control their assets. If your senior is divorced, a widow, or a widower and isn't comfortable giving their assets away, then Medicaid estate planning is not appropriate for them. It also does not make sense for wealthy individuals with substantial assets.

It also doesn't work well for:

- Someone who has never been married or has no intended heirs

- Someone without a strong family support system

- Someone who is mentally incompetent unless adequate legal documents are in place

Three Things You Should Know About Medicaid Estate Planning

In seeking a Medicaid solution, you should know:

- There *is* help available.

- You *don't* have to spend everything.

- You *can* find someone who knows what they're doing!

Sometimes people think their case is simple enough to handle on their own. But honest mistakes can cost you a small fortune. The fees of a qualified Medicaid estate planner are well worth the expense.

Here are some other things to keep in mind:

- Inexperienced advisors can really cost you.

- Information on the internet can be dangerously out of date or inaccurate.

- Medicaid rules change frequently — work with someone in the know.

- Misinformation is everywhere: nursing home staff and Medicaid employees. Many speak with great certainty when they shouldn't.

- Don't expect nursing home intake staff to know Medicaid law.

- Don't expect a store-bought or online power-of-attorney to work for you. Invest in a knowledgeable attorney.

- Be careful about giving away your assets. You may face such risks as squandering, lawsuits, bankruptcy, divorce and bad business deals.

Three Examples

Chances are these scenarios will sound familiar to you. I share them with you to illustrate the huge advantage of hiring an expert to guide your pursuit of eldercare funding.

Example #1

An 81-year-old woman is entering a nursing home. Along with her 79-year-old husband, their combined monthly income is $2,324, but her long-term care costs are $4,800. This means they have a negative cash flow of $2,500 per month — more than they earn.

Their total countable assets are $33,000, and their home is worth $89,000. He decided to put it on the market. Their Medicaid estate planner advised him that he didn't need to sell the home and to take it off the market. This means he can live in his own home instead of moving into a less-desirable apartment.

Example #2

A 63-year-old woman had developed Alzheimer's disease very early in life. Her 66-year-old husband had been caring for her on his own for 20 years. He's given all his money to his daughter in an attempt to qualify for Medicaid. His Medicaid estate planner advised him to unwind that and to follow the existing expansion provisions, so the money was protected. In this case the timing of the return of his money from the daughter in relation to the wife's nursing home placement was critical.

They had a monthly income of $2,023 and a negative cash flow of $4,300. The planner used those special protections to protect every penny the husband had. He's got another 20 years of living— had he applied to Medicaid on his own, he would have been denied and may have never been able to place his wife in a nursing home. But, by working with a planner, he was able to protect his house and his assets.

Example #3

Consider an older couple: the husband is 72 years old, and the wife is 73. The husband is going to a nursing home. Their Texas home is worth $350,000, and they had assets worth $155,000. Their income was $2,200 a month.

The house has a $325,000 note, and their credit cards are maxed out. The wife is trying to maintain the 6-bedroom home, pay for her husband's $6,000 monthly nursing home costs and pay the mortgage. They have $152,000 of illiquid assets and only $3,000 in the bank.

A Medicaid Estate planner would likely be able to get her qualified with Medicaid by proving their assets were inaccessible. Medicaid declares that once assets are established, you are not allowed to exceed that amount ever. If her bank account ever exceeded that $3,000–even just for a day—she'd be disqualified. She really had to keep an eye on that amount like a hawk to make sure she didn't go over the limit.

This last case is a great example of why you should work closely with a fully-qualified and experienced Medicaid estate planner. Here are three more things to look for in a Medicaid Planner:

- **Specialization:** Make sure they have extensive experience with Medicaid estate planning

- **Excellent communication skills:** Avoid jargon-speakers and fast-talkers; opt for a planner that takes the time to explain the process and your options.

- **Trustworthiness:** As with any other professional you hire for your eldercare needs, listen to your intuition and only hire someone you trust.

Special Thanks

A special thanks goes to Martin "Mr. Elder Care" Sabel for his expertise in the complex world of Medicaid planning. Martin is located in Houston, Texas and can be reach via his contact information below.

Martin Sabel, Elder Care Strategist
The Elder Law Firm of Mulder and Freedman
4545 Mount Vernon
Houston, Texas 77006
Phone: 713-306-5002

Need a Provider in Your State?

Inside Elder Care maintains a Medicaid planning providers nationwide. For a list of Medicaid planning providers in your state, visit www.insideeldercare.com/medicaid-planning

EIGHT

WRAPPING IT ALL UP

Paying for senior care can be a frustrating and tiring challenge in your life. Every situation is slightly different, and everyone has different needs for their loved ones. While there certainly is no panacea for solving these challenges, you do have options.

The more you know about the different funding options, the more successful you will be in finding a solution that works for you. The more options you uncover, the less likely you are to be stressed-out.

As you work through this challenge in your life, be diligent and determined. Don't be afraid to ask questions. Whomever you choose to assist you with this planning, remember that they are providing you a service. You are the customer and have the right to ask as many questions as you want, shop around to as many providers as you want and even change your mind at the last minute.

In closing, I would love to hear about your journey and any interesting options you uncover. Please don't be a stranger—I'm always available at ryan@insideeldercare.com.

Good luck!

www.ingramcontent.com/pod-product-compliance
Lightning Source LLC
Chambersburg PA
CBHW062106280526
45788CB00003B/1364